William Cadogan

A dissertation on the gout and all chronic diseases, jointly considered, as proceeding from the same causes:

What those causes are; and a rational and natural method of cure

proposed; addressed to all invalids

William Cadogan

A dissertation on the gout and all chronic diseases, jointly considered, as proceeding from the same causes:
What those causes are; and a rational and natural method of cure proposed; addressed to all invalids

ISBN/EAN: 9783337731342

Printed in Europe, USA, Canada, Australia, Japan

Cover: Foto ©ninafisch / pixelio.de

More available books at **www.hansebooks.com**

U T,

ISEASES,

Y. CONSIDERED,

g from the fame CAU

ſe CAUSES are

A N D

METHOD of CURE
ſed.

Addreſſed all INVALIDS.

By WILLIAM CADOGAN,

FELLOW of the COLLEGE of PHYSICIANS.

THE TENTH EDITION.

Quod petis in te eſt.

LONDON, Printed:
BOSTON: Re-printed for HENRY KNOX, in
Cornhill, MDCCLXXII.

TO enjoy good health is better than to command the world, fays a celebrated practical philofo-pher*, who underftood the ufe and value of life and health better than moft men ; for in exile,with a fmall income, and no very good conftitution, he cultivated an uncommon length of days into a rational feries of pleafures ; and what is much more, an uninter-rupted courfe of happinefs. But, as far as I can find, he was almoft the only man that did fo. The generality of men feem to me not to beftow a tho't upon either, till it be too late to reap the benefit of their conviction ; fo that health, like time, becomes valuable only when it is loft; and we can no longer think of it but with retrofpect and regret.

That men in good health, the young and gay in their career, fhould be negligent of it, or abufe it, refufing to ftop and liften to, or take warning from others, is no great wonder ; but it is very furprizing that mankind in general fhould be miftaken and miflead forever in the fame perpetual round of fruit-lefs attempts to repair and eftablifh it ; not the ig-norant vulgar only, but the fenfible the judicious, men of parts, and knowledge in other things, in this cafe equally blind, fhould purfue, with the fame vain hope, after repeated difappointments, the thoufand and ten thoufand idle arts and tricks of medication and quackery ; never once lifting their eyes up to

* St. Evremond.

Nature, or confulting her book, open as it lies for the perufal, conviction and benefit of all.

Some induftrious men, fancying that whatever is valuable muft lie deep, have, with the greateft alacrity in finking, plunged into the immenfe abyfs of ancient, Greek, Roman and Arabic learning, in hopes to find good precepts of health, and fure remedy for difeafe. But after all their pioneering into endlefs heaps of rubbifh, what have they found at laft but this ? That in natural philofophy fome of the ancients were very ingenious in gueffing wrong; for guefs was all they did ; they never ftudied Nature at all, they made no experiments, and therefore knew nothing of her ; but either blindly followed or combated each others opinions : fchool againft fchool, and fect againft fect, waged equal and endlefs war. In the art of phyfic it was impoffible for them to know much; for before our immortal HARVEY's difcovery of the circulation, there could be no phyfiology at all, nor any knowledge either of the internal ftructure or action of any one part of the body. Before the juftly celebrated ASELLIUS and PEQUET there could be no idea of nourifhment ; nor was it known how our food paffed into the blood, whether it went there or not, or what became of it. But now, fince thefe lights have fhone in upon us, all the ancient conjectures, reafonings, and fyftems, muft vanifh like morning clouds before the fun. Befides all this, there are fome of our difeafes which the ancients had not, nor have we all theirs : fome few, and very few ufeful, difcoveries they made in medicine, which have defcended to us, and with fome late tricks in chemiftry are the chief foundation of modern quackery. Thus have men of deep learning, if the knowledge of ancient errors can be called fo, funk far out of fight of truth, which in things of general ufe and neceffity, particularly the health of mankind, lies moft commonly upon the furface.

It has been of great differvice, as well as difcredit to the art of Phyfic, and every fair practifer of it, that men's expectations have been raifed by the ignorant and prefuming, or the difhoneft and artful, to hope for too much from it, more than it ever did or can do. Refpite and relief may be had in moft chronic cafes ; remedy, I fear but in very few, if it be expected from art alone. But a fkilful and honeft Phyfician (unlefs he be fent for too late and difmiffed too foon, which is generally the cafe) will employ thofe intervals of relief to introduce the powers of life and nature to act for themfelves, and infenfibly withdrawing all his medicines, and watching carefully over his patient's whole conduct, leave him confirmed, from conviction of their neceffity, in fuch good and falutary habits, as cannot fail to eftablifh his health for life.

Poffibly, if men were better informed of the real caufes of their difeafes, they might be lefs unreafonable in their demands, and learn to be contented with prefent relief ; fubmitting with patience to that plan of life which alone can lead them to, and preferve them in, permanent health. With this view of engaging men's attention to their own happinefs, and undeceiving them in their vain and groundlefs hopes of remedy, and diverting them from the delufions of art to the realities of nature, I have ventured to publifh the following Differtation ; which

I muſt beg the reader to conſider as, what it really is, a haſty extract of a much larger work, intended to take in the whole circle of Chronic Diſeaſes, here comprehended only in their repreſentative the Gout. If what I have ſaid may ſeem to want farther illuſtration, or more demonſtrative proof, he will look upon it only as a ſketch to furniſh hints for his own thoughts and reflections, either to improve mine or reject them entirely, as may ſeem good unto him. If he thinks, from what I have ſaid here, or in the *brochure* itſelf, that I mean to impeach the practice of phyſic in general ; I ſay, that it is not my intention. I would decry all quacks, from Æſculapius to the preſent, either as ignorant fools, or ſelf-convicted impoſtors, advertiſing daily lies ; whether mounted on ſtages, or riding in chariots. But the art of phyſic fairly and honeſtly practiſed I honour as the firſt of profeſſions, comprehending the moſt uſeful, the moſt extenſive and univerſal knowledge of nature. I think a real Phyſician the moſt liberal of characters upon earth ; by which I do not mean every Doctor that goes about taking guineas, but him who will neither flatter the great nor deceive the ignorant, and who would prefer the ſatisfaction of making one invalid a healthy man, to the wealth of *Radcliff* or the vogue of *Ward*. But there is an evil ſpirit of quackery gone forth, that has poſſeſſed all orders of men among us. I would lay it if I could, together with every demon of ſuperſtition, fraud, and error, and reſtore the world to truth and nature.

George-Street, Hanover-Square,
Nov. 20. 1771.

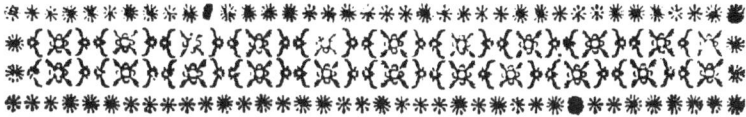

A

DISSERTATION

ON THE

G O U T, &c.

H OWEVER common it may be for men that suffer to complain of the evils of life, as the unavoidable lot of humanity; would they stop but for a moment to consider them in the light of reason and philosophy, they would find little or no foundation for them in nature; but that every man was the real author of all or most of his own miseries. Whatever doubts may be entertained of moral evils, the natural, for the most part, such as bodily infirmity, sickness, and pain; all that class of complaints which the learned call chronic diseases, we most undoubtedly bring upon ourselves by our own indulgencies, excesses, or mistaken habits of life; or by suffering our ill-conducted passions to lead us astray or disturb our peace of mind. Whatever notions men have been taught or have received of other caufes, fuch as accidental colds, or particularities of conftitution, this or that thing difagreeing or furfeiting, &c. thefe are too trifling to produce difeafes that commonly laft for life : there muft be fomething more fubftantial, fomething more conftant and parmanent in our daily habits, to produce fuch inveterate evils. Though if you read authors or confult practitioners, what do you find, but that you have taken cold, though you know not how, or that your complaints are gouty, rheumatic, bilious, nervous, &c. ? words that fatisfy, though they give no kind of idea, and feem to have gained credit and affent only by the politenefs of phyficians, who, while they are taking their patients money, are too well bred to tell them difagreeable truths, and that it is by there own faults they are ill. To enquire a little further into this matter may be well worth our trouble ; the tafk feems to have been left for me, and I will perform it moft fincerely.

I have long had it in my mind to write upon chronic difeafes in general, in the hope of giving mankind, what moft affuredly they have never yet had, a few rational ideas about them ; thinking that, if the true original caufes of them were fully and fairly fet forth, men could not be fo capitally miftaken to impute them, as they do, to the falfe and imaginary, and therefore apply falfe and imaginary remedies ; nor think that the general health of mankind were to be overfet by every trifle, and the recovery of it lay hid in a few drops or powders of any kind. Did they better underftand the

nature of chronic difeafes in general, and whence
they proceed, they could not be fo unreafonable to
think they might live as they lift with impunity,
expecting repeated remedy from art ; or, did they
know any thing of the nature of medicine, they
would find that, though fits of pain have been relieved, or ficknefs cured by it for a time, the eftab-
lifhment of health is a very different thing, depending upon other powers and principles : the firft
may be and often is done by medicine,the other never. That their opinion of medicine is vain and
ridiculous muft appear, I think, very evidently to
any one who recollects that the art of phyfic has
now been practifed, more or lefs regularly, above
two thoufand years ; and moft affuredly there is not
yet difcovered any one certain remedy for any difeafe. Ought not this to make us fufpect that there
is no fuch thing ? How can it be, when different
degrees of the very fame difeafe require various
means and methods, and the fame thing that in one
degree would relieve, or perhaps cure, in another
might kill ? It is by plan, by regimen, and fucceffive
intention, that difeafes muft be cured, when they
are curable ; or relieved and palliated when they
are not. The fkilful in medicine, and learned in
nature, know well that health is not to be eftablifhed by medicine ; for it's effects are but momentary,
and the frequent repetition of it deftructive to the
ftrongeft frames ; that if it is to be reftored, it muft
be by gently calling forth the powers of the body
to act for themfelves, introducing gradually a little
more and more activity, chofen diet, and, above all,
peace of mind, changing intirely that courfe of life

which firſt brought on the diſeaſe : medicine co-operating a little. That this is the truth, all who know any thing of nature or art muſt know : and I may ſafely take upon me to ſay, that, though I firmly believe health may be reſtored in moſt caſes that are not abſolutely mortal, I am very ſure that no invalid was ever made a healthy man by the mere power of medicine. If this be the caſe, how muſt the initiated, according as their humanity is touched, either laugh at or pity the poor fooliſh world, ſurrendering at diſcretion to the moſt ignorant of quacks, pretending to infallible remedies which are not in nature. But what is ſtill more ridiculous, the patients themſelves are often ſo aſhamed to own they have been deluded, that they favor the cheat, by pretending to relief which they never felt.

I have collected a few materials for this work, which I intend to put in order, as ſoon as I can find time and induſtry enough to ſet about it in earneſt ; and, if I can finiſh it to my own ſatisfaction, perhaps I may ſome time or other trouble the world with it. At preſent I think myſelf particularly called upon to ſay ſomething of the gout, as that diſeaſe was to make a conſiderable part of my plan ; and, as I ſee now ſo many, and hear of more, who are throwing away, not only their money very fooliſhly, but, as I verily believe, the future health of their lives alſo, in hopes of a medical cure for it, to ſhew that ſuch hopes are chimerical, and contradictory to every idea of true philoſophy and common ſenſe.

I fhall therefore take a few extracts from this ge; neral plan, fufficient to fhew the real original caufes of all chronic difeafes ; which, though they have been multiplied without end, and numberlefs caufes been affigned them, are certainly not many, and their firft caufes very few. I think they may very fairly be reduced to thefe three : Indolence, in temperance, and Vexation.

From one or more of thefe three caufes, I have undertaken to prove that all or moft chronic difeafes are produced ; for different difeafes may have the fame original caufe, the difference proceeding from the various degrees of ftrength and vigor in bodies ; fo that what would be gout in one, in another might be rheumatifm, ftone, colic, jaundice, palfy, &c. The gout is manifeftly and I think confeffedly, a difeafe of the beft conftitution, and may therefore fairly ftand as a reprefentative of all the reft : as fuch I fhall confider it for the prefent, and fpeak of thefe caufes in their order : but it may be neceffary to fay a word or two of the gout itfelf before we enquire into its caufe.

The gout is fo common a difeafe, that there is fcarcely a man in the world, whether he has had it or not, but thinks he knows perfectly what it is. So does a cook-maid think fhe knows what fire is as well as Sir JfaacNewton. It may therefore feem needlefs at prefent to trouble ourfelves about a definition, to fay what it is : but I will venture to fay what I am perfuaded it is not, though contrary to the general opinion. It is not hereditary, it is not periodical, and it is not incurable.

If it were hereditary, it would be neceffarily tranfmitted from father to fon, and no man whofe father had it could poffibly be free from it : but this is not the cafe, there are many inftances to the contrary : it is therefore not neceffarily fo ; but the father's having it inclines or difpofes the fon to it. This is the *caufa proegumena* or *prædifponent* of the learned, which of itfelf never produced any effect at all ; there muft be joined the *caufa procatarctica*, or active efficient caufe, that is, our own intemperance or miftaken habit of life, to produce it ; and accordingly, as this operates more or lefs, fo will the gout be. Our parents undoubtedly give us conftitutions fimilar to their own, and, if we live in the fame manner they did, we fhall very probably be troubled with the fame difeafes ; but this by no means proves them to be hereditary : it is what we do ourfelves that will either bring them on, or keep us free.

If it were hereditary, it would appear in infancy and in women, which in general it does not. I may be told of fome women who have had it. I believe never very young, nor till they had contributed to it themfelves ; for women, as well as men, may a-bufe a good conftitution. I have heard likewife of a boy or two out of a million that had it, or fomething like it ; but thefe boys had been fuffered to fip wine very early, and been fed and indulged every way moft unwholefomely.

Thofe, who infift that the gout is hereditary, be-caufe they think they fee it fo fometimes, muft argue very inconclufively ; for if we compute the number of children who have it not, and women who have it not, together with all thofe active and temperate men who are free from it, though born of gouty parents ; the proportion will be found at leaft a hundred to one againft that opinion. And furely I have a greater right from all thefe inftances to fay that it is not hereditary, then they have from a few to contend that it is. What is all this, but to pronounce a difeafe hereditary, and prove it by faying that it is fometimes fo, but oftener not fo ? Can there be a greater abfurdity.

Some men obferving, in the circle of their acquaintance, the children of gouty parents afflicted with the gout, and often very early in life, though they are what they call temperate, conclude, not unnaturally, that the difeafe muft be parental, and unavoidably transfufed into their conftitutions. If this were the cafe, it muft be for ever incurable, and the fins of the father vifited upon the children not only of three or four but endlefs generations to come. Difeafes really hereditary, I fear, are never cured by any art or method whatever, as is but too true in the cafes of fcrophula and madnefs, and difeafes of taint or infection, and maleformation. But here lies the error, their idea of temperance is by on means juft * : for fome men require a greater degree, a ftricter mode of it than others, to be kept in good health. I make no doubt but if the lives thefe gouty defcendants lead were clofely inquired into by

* See Chapter of Intemperance, p. 41.

real phyficians, they would be found to commit many errors, and to fin often againſt nature's law of temperance, or to want that conſtant peace of mind or regular activity of body which are as neceſſary as temperance, not only to keep off the gout, but to preferve health in general; aud thus it will appear at laſt that they have contributed to it more than their parents.

If the gout be a difeafe of indigeſtion, and therefore of our own acquiring, we muſt reafon very ill, or rather not reafon at all, when we fay it is hereditary; for furely no man will fay that indigeſtion is hereditary, any more than intemperance. There are whole nations of active people knowing no luxury, who for ages have been free from it, but have it now fince the Europeans have brought them wine and fpirits.

If the gout be thought hereditary becaufe it is incurable by medicine, the fame may be faid of every other chronic difeafe, none of which ever are cured by it, I mean, fo as not to return again. When was there a man who, having had one fit of rheumatifm, ſtone, colic, &c. however happily relieved by art for a time, had it not again and again, or fomething worfe in the place of it; till he became a confirmed invalid, and died long before his time, unlefs fome very remarkable alteration took place in the courfe of his life to confirm his health? So it is in the gout : a man gets a fit of it, and by abſtinence, patience, time and nature, the crude acrimony producing it is fubdued and exhauſted, and he is relieved for that time ; (he might be fo much fooner, and very fafely too, by the affiftance of art judicioufly employed) : he recovers however, and in a few months is taken again. Why ? Not from any thing inherent in his conftitution, but becaufe he returned to his former habit of life that produced it at firft, and will for ever produce it, while the ftrength of his body lafts.

The truth is, we breed it at firft, we renew it again and again, and bring it on ourfelves by our own miftakes or faults, which we would fain excufe by throwing them back upon our parents, that our complaints may be more juftly founded. And as bankrupts, undone by idlenefs and extravagance, for ever plead loffes and misfortunes ; fo do we inheritance, to exculpate ourfelves.

It is natural enough for thofe who believe the gout hereditary to think it alfo periodical, as if fomething innate and inherent in our conftitutions produced it at certain times : but this is a great miftake ; for, if it were periodical, it muft be regularly fo. The only periodical difeafe I know is the intermittent fever, which, till it be diftrubed by the bark or any other febrifuge, is as regular as a good clock. The returns of the gout are always very uncertain, according to the quantity or quality of accumulated indigeftion within, and the ftrength of our bodies.

I come now to fhew that the gout is not incurable. If by the cure of it be meant the adminiftering a pill or a powder, or medicine of any kind to do it, I fear it is and ever will be incurable. It has been long and often attempted in vain, from the origin of phyfic to this day, from the firft quack to the prefent. Indeed there is a moft glaring abfurdity at firft fight, that muft ftop any man of common fenfe, who has the leaft infight into nature, or knowledge of the human frame : for, if the gout be the neceffary effect of intemperance, as I hope to fhew very evidently that it is, a medicine to cure it muft be fomething that will enable a man to bear the daily intemperance of his future life unhurt by the gout or any other difeafe ; that is, fomething given now that will take away the effect of a future caufe. As well might a medicine be given now to prevent a man's breaking his leg or his neck feven years hence. One would think the utmoft that any rational man could expect from medicine was, that it fhould have power to relieve and remove prefent diforders, leaving the body quite free, without pretending to infure it from future injuries. Here lies the error : men think the gout to be fomething latent in the body now, which, once well eradicated, would never return ; not fufpecting it to be no more than each day's indigeftion accumulated to a certain pitch, that, as long as the vigor of life lafts, always brings on every fit, which once well over, the man has no more gout, nor feeds of gout in him, than he who never had it ; and, if he did not breed it again, moft certainly would never have it again. A proof of this is, that the gout has been often cured by a milk diet, which, as long as it lasted, has generally kept the patient free. But this method of cure I cannot approve, becaufe it relaxes and enervates the man, and does not fufficiently fupport the health and vigour of his body.

Though I think the gout incurable by medicine, it is fo far from being incurable in its nature, that I am firmly perfuaded it may be more eafily and more perfectly cured than almoft any other chronic difeafe; and this is another ftrong argument that proves it not hereditary. My reafon is, that it is confeffedly a difeafe of the ftrongeft and beft conftitution relieving itfelf by throwing off harfh and bad humors from the vitals, and out of the blood upon the extremities, where they do leaft harm to the powers and principles of life and health; and as thefe humors can be nothing more than the daily accumulations of indigeftion, if a man can live without breeding conftantly this indigefted acrimony, he may moft undoubtedly live free, not only from the gout, but every other chronic difeafe alfo. And that he may live fo, not in a perpetual ftate of mortification and felf-denial, but with great eafe and comfort to himfelf, in the trueft, moft philofophic luxury, I fhall endeavour to prove, I hope to the fatisfaction of all thinking, reafonable men.

I have faid, that Indolence, Intemperence, and Vexation, are the original caufes of all or moft of our chronic difeafes: perhaps a few accidents muft be excepted, to which the ftrongeft and healthieft

are moft liable ; and the effects of fevers not happily ended ; and which I except, to obviate all cavil
and difpute with the men of art. I believe, to every
confiderate man, whofe eyes have been opened fo
as to give the leaft infight into nature, the truth of
this propofition will be fo felf-evident, that he muft
inftantly perceive it ; and every invalid that will be
candid enough to do it, may fairly trace all his complaints up to one or other of thefe caufes. But it
may require fome explanation to the generality of
men, who are fo fhort-fighted as never to look back
or forward far beyond the ken of their nofe, and
therefore never fee either diftant caufes or effects ;
and when they are fick feldom enquire more than
for fome cold or furfeit of yefterday, and to fome
fuch trifling caufe impute difeafes that laft for life.
An accidental cold or even debauch that happens
but feldom can have no fuch effect ; and men
otherwife healthly, living in good habits, foon get
rid of both. It is the conftant courfe of life we lead,
what we do, or neglect to do, habitualy every day,
that if right eftablifhes our health, if wrong, makes
us invalids for life.

Men ignorant of the ways of nature in the pro-
duction and fupport of animals, not knowing what
fhe requires to preferve them in health and vigour
to their utmoft period, have conceived very ftrange
and moft affuredly very falfe ideas of difeafes in
general, and feem to think every difeafe a diftinct
kind of being or thing, and that there are medicines
oppofed to each, that will certainly remove and cure

it. This makes them fo folicitous to know the name of their complaint, which once afcertained, they think the remedy not far off. Poor men ! Is not the gout fufficiently diftinguifhed ? But where is the remedy ? Certainly not in the precarious fkill of prefcribing doctors, or the fecret of ignorant and enterprizing quacks. They fancy too that there is great variety of conftitution, with difeafes unavoidable peculiar to each : that certain times of life muft produce many, and that it is impoffible to grow old without ficknefs of fome kind or other. There is certainly no foundation in nature for any of thefe opinions, nor is there any real effential difference of conftitution, but of ftrong or weak, and this is produced more by habit than nature. The ftrong by bad habits will become weaker, and by good the weak ftronger. But the moft delicate frames may be as healthy as the ftrongeft, for the fame reafon that a fquirrel may be as healthy as an elephant. There is no difeafe neceffarily peculiar to any time of life, however the changes into the different ftages of it may effect the valetudinary. And it is poffible for men to live to great age without any difeafe at all, for many have lived to upwards of an hundred with uninterrupted health.

Not from the natural defects of our conftitutions therefore, but the abufe of them, proceed all our chronic difeafes. That is, from Indolence, Intemperance, or Vexation. Let us now proceed to enquire what muft be the neceffary effect of one or more of thefe caufes acting daily upon the body ;

whether in the ftrongeft and moft vigorous frames it muft not be the gout ; in weaker, rheumatifm, colic, ftone, palfy, &c. or any, or all of the nervous and hyfterical clafs.

First, of Indolence, by which I do not mean infenfibility, but an inactive habit of life, taking the word in the general common fenfe it is now ufed.

Of INDOLENCE.

IT feems to have been the defign of Providence that all men fhould labor, every one for himfelf. That fome are rich enough to purchafe the ftrength and activity of others is a mere accident with regard to individuals, in which the care of Providence appears to be no otherwife concerned, than having unequally diftributed thofe powers and abilities by which active and fiery fpirits rife uppermoft to preferve the harmony of fubordination, without which fociety could never exift. The rich and great have fo far forgot this firft principle of nature, that they renounce all bodily labor as unworthy their condition, and are either too lazy or too inattentive to fubftitute exercife inftead of it : thus facrificing health to indulgence and dignity, they do not enjoy thofe advantages their fuperior ftations and fortunes give them ; but in happinefs fall often below the laboring hind. I remember to have feen a very ingenious little book upon the origin of evil, in which labor is confidered as a great evil. The agreeable author muft furely

mean when it's exceffive, and urged on the wearing
and wafting the body ; for in general it is the firft
principle of good to mankind, and to none more
than the laborious themfelves. Does he mean that it
would be better for us all, did the earth fpontaneoufly bring forth her fruits in fuch abundance, that
we fhould no more labor or contend for them than
we do for the air, and have nothing to do but bafk
in eafe, and riot in enjoyment ? If fo I can by no
means agree with him ; for foon, very foon, in fuch a
ftate of things, there would not be one healthy man
upon the earth, and the whole race muft quickly
perifh. Indeed I am afraid, notwithftanding all
our unreafonable and unphilofophical complainings,
the utmoft wit of man cannot remove the leaft evil
out of nature, without taking with it all the good.
But begging pardon for this little digreffion, and
to come back to my own purpofe, I think he had
been nearer the truth, had he put indolence in its
ftead, which is a fource of great evil. Nothing under-
mines the foundation of all our happinefs, the health
and vigor of the body, like it, or lays fuch a train
of difeafes to come. But I muft endeavor to fhew
in what manner.

It is upon the minuteft and almoft invifible parts
of the body our beft health, ftrength, and fpirits depend : thefe fine parts, commonly called capillaries,
are little pipes or tubes, the extended continuations
of the larger blood veffels, through which the fineft
parts of the blood muft conftantly pafs, not only to
keep thefe very fmall channels always free and open,
but alfo that the particles of the blood may in their

paſſage be attenuated, broken, and rubbed into globules perfectly ſmooth and round, and eaſily di- viſible in ſtill leſs and leſs, till they eſcape the ſight aſſiſted even by the microſcope ; which gives ocular demonſtration of this moſt amazingly minute circula- tion. I have obſerved myſelf, and any curious pa- tient man may ſee with a good microſcope, in the pellucid membrane of any living animal, this ſur- prizing minuteneſs. He may ſelect and obſerve one ſingle veſſel, the ſmalleſt of thoſe that convey red blood, many of which would not equal the ſmalleſt hair in ſize, through which the blood may be ſeen paſſing, not like a fluid, but a number of little red ſo- lid balls puſhing one another on till they come to the extremity or ramification of the veſſel where it divides into two ſtill leſs. There the firſt globule, ſtopping a little, and recoiling, is puſhed on again till it divides into two, and, loſing its red colour, paſſes on in the ſmaller pipes fitted only to receive the ſerum ; which undergoes the ſame circulation till it be refined into lymph, and this into ſtill finer flu- ids ; which, being thus prepared, eſcape into a ſub- tility beyond all poſſible obſervation. Now the ſtrength of the heart and arteries alone, in a ſeden- tary courſe of life, is by no means ſufficient to keep up and perpetuate this motion through theſe capila- ries, but requires the aſſiſtance and joint force of all the muſcles of the body to act by intervals, compreſs the veins, propel and accelerate the circulation of the whole maſs of blood, in order to force and clear theſe pipes, and to triturate, cribrate, and purify the fluid paſſing through, forming every particle of it

into a perfect globule, which is the form all the a-
toms of matter muſt take from much agitation.
Without this extraordinary occaſional aid, the little
veſſels would, by their natural elaſticity, cloſe up into fibres, or be obſtructed by rough angular particles
ſticking in them, and ſtopping all paſſage. Num-
berleſs evils of the chronic kind, eſpecially all nervous diſeaſes, owe their origin to this cauſe alone.
Accordingly we ſee moſt of thoſe who have lived for
any time in a ſtate of indolence, grow emaciated and
pale by the drying up of theſe fine veſſels ; or, if
they happen to be of a lax habit, having a good appetite, and nothing to vex them, they may be loaded
with fat ; but they grow pale withal, many of thoſe
fine pipes being neverthelefs cloſed up ; ſo that
they appear bloated, and their fat unwholſome,
having much leſs blood in their veins than thinner
people. Hence we may learn why theſe languid
pale perſons upon the leaſt motion become faint and
breathleſs, the blood hurrying through the larger
veſſels yet free, and, like a crowd obſtructing its own
paſſage, cauſing a dangerous ſuffocation. Or, if
they have not been long in this ſtate, nor the capillaries quite cloſed, they glow, eſpecially young wo-,
men, with a momentary red, the fine veſſels being
for that time expanded. Thus inactivity firſt forms
obſtructions in theſe exquiſitely fine parts, upon
which the health and vigor both of body and mind
depend entirely, and lays the foundation of many
diſeaſes to come ; which other concomitant circum-
ſtances, ſuch as a violent cold, exceſs of any kind,

infection from without, or a particular difpofition of
the body within, make often fatal to many in this
habit of life ; and which the induftrious and active
never feel.

Now I would afk any reafonable perfon, capable
of confidering this operation of nature with the leaft
glimmering of philofophy, or even the attention of
common fenfe, and moft affuredly it concerns every
man to confider it well, whether he can conceive it
poffible to fubftitute any medicine to be fwallowed,
that fhall act upon the blood and veffels like the
joint force of all the mufcles of the body, acting and
reacting occafionally in a regular courfe of moderate
daily labor or exercife.   Unlefs this can be done, I
will venture to pronounce that there is no fuch thing
as a lafting cure, either for the gout or any other
chronic difeafe.   Yes, Sir, fays a common practi-
tioner, cordials, volatiles, bracers, ftrengtheners,
will do this, will keep up an increafed circulation.
Poffibly they may for a few hours, by doing mifchief
for many days : but their action foon fubfides, and
the ftimulus ceafes ; they muft therefore be repeated and repeated for life.   Woe be to him that takes
them,& to him that leaves them off,unlefsit be done
with great judgment.   While they act, they coagu-
late the juices and corrupt the whole mafs of blood ;
and when omitted, the patient muft feel all the lan-
guors and horrors of a crapulary fever after repeated
debauch ; and muft have recourfe to them again and
again, like a dram-drinker, who cannot bear his

exiſtence but in a ſtate of intoxication. No, art can never come up to nature in this moſt ſalutary of all her operations.

But theſe obſtructions from crude particles of the blood, and this inanition of the capillaries, are not all the evils produced by indolence. That ſprightly vigor and alacrity of health which we feel and enjoy in an active courſe of life, that zeſt in apetite, and refreſhment after eating, which ſated luxury ſeeks in vain from art, is owing wholly to new blood made every day from freſh food prepared and diſtributed by the joint action of all the parts of the body. No man can have theſe delightful ſenſations who lives two days with the ſame blood, but muſt be languid and ſpiritleſs. To introduce new juices the old muſt be firſt thrown off, or there will be no room, there will be too great a plethora or fulneſs ; the firſt cauſe of diſeaſe in many caſes. In a ſtate of inactivity the old humors paſs off ſo ſlowly, the inſenſible perſpiration is ſo inconſiderable, that there is no void to be filled ; conſequently by degrees the appetite, which is the laſt thing that decays, that is, the deſire of ſupply, muſt daily diminiſh, and at laſt be totally loſt. Here art can do wonders ; it can procure evacuations ; we can bleed, purge, and vomit ; but then, to do any good by theſe, the caſe muſt be recent, before the humors are vitiated by too long a ſtay in the body, which will be the caſe very ſoon, for they are all in a periſhable ſtate, which makes their daily renewal ſo eſſentially neceſſary to health : but theſe theſe artificial evacuations diſcharge all alike ; the new, the middle, and the old juices; that is, the chyle, the blood, the ferum, and lymph; and by this indifcriminate action make ftrange confufion in thofe that remain; whereas in nature's courfe there is a conftant regular tranfmutation and fucceffion from one ftate to another; that is, from chyle into blood, and blood into ferum, ferum into lymph, and fo on, till they are all in their turn, having done their office in various fhapes, elaborated and ground to fuch a minute fubtility and finenefs, that, like wave impelling wave, they fucceffively pafs off in the vapor of infenfible perfpiration. In a ftate of indolence they do not pafs off either fo foon or fo regularly as they ought, becaufe there is not motion, nor confequently heat enough to throw off the vapor : they lodge in the body too long, grow putrid, acrimonious, and hurtful many ways, like the matter formed in an ulcer, which, while it is yet fweet, is more healing than any balfam the furgeon can apply; but, when confined, it foon becomes corrofive, and like a cauftic eats it's way all round in fiftulas to find vent. This fhews the virulent acrimony of thefe confined and ftagnating humors : hence the breath and perfpiration, what there is of it occafionly, of indolent people is never fweet; and hence in jails, where thefe noxious vapors are collected and condenfed from crouded wretches languifhing in indolence, very malignant and peftilential fevers arife.

Perpetual blifters have been often thought, and fometimes found, to be ferviceable in draining off fome of the fuperfluous juices before they are much corrupted, and making, by a faint refemblance of nature's action, a little more room for new : and it is for this reason they do any good at all, by increasing the general circulation, and forcing off a few of of those humors that had circulated too long in the body, and were becoming acrid : for the quantity they discharge is so trifling, that there could be no physiology, nor even common sense, in supposing the evacution to be the benefit procured. By a vomit or a purge the discharge is a hundred fold more, but the good obtained not always so great, because by these the humors are indiscriminately thrown off, & much more of the new than the old. Many have used frequent bleeding to renew their blood, and I have known it answer very well to some, especially old people who had been long accustomed to it, whom it preserved to great age : but then it must be begun in time, before the whole mass of humors be vitiated, and continued for life. Is it not strange that men should seek and prefer these violent artificial methods to the simple, easy, pleasant, and constant action of nature, and chuse rather to take a vomit or a purge than a walk, and wear a perpetual blister than make the least use of their limbs ?

Thus indolence must inevitably lay the foundation of general disease, and according to the constitution and a few concomitant circumstances will be the kind of the disease : in the very best it may be gout or rheumatism ; in the weaker habits colic, jaundice, palsy, stone, &c. with all of the hysterical & hypochondriacal class. In vain have ingenious men of reading and study, mental labor and fedentary life, who are more fubject to difeafe in general than the gay and thoughtlefs, endeavored to obviate the evil by abftinence, an excellent means of remedy in many cafes, and which few practife but true philofophers, who are not the moft likely to want it. But yet even they do not find it anfwer, and for the reafons which I have juft given ; that we can- not live two days in health and fpirits with the fame blood ; there muft be a new daily fupply of that ethe- real part of our food called up to the brain to fup- port its own, as well as the labor of the whole body. By this I mean the moft elaborated, refined parts of all our juices, which conftantly repairs and nourifhes the fmalleft veffels and fibres ; whether I may be allowed to call it animal fpirits or not, is not material. Whenever this æther fails, we muft neceffarily feel langour and laffitude both of body and mind : with this difference, that in wearinefs of the limbs from much action the lees and coarfer parts are thrown off alfo, and the firft meal and firft fleep foon fupplies the defect. In mental labor the feculence remains to obftruct all appetite ; there is no room, and there- fore no call for fupply ; the whole man fuffers and finks.

Of INTEMPERANCE.

I COME now to fpeak of Intemperance ; for Indolence, blunting all our fenfations, natu- rally leads us to intemperance : we want the whip and fpur of luxury to excite our jaded appetites.

There is no enduring the perpetual moping languor of indolence : we fly to the ſtimulating ſenſualities of the table and the bottle, friend provokes friend to exceed, and accumulate one evil upon another ; a joyous momentary relief is obtained, to be paid for ſeverely ſoon after ; the next morning our horrors increaſe, and in this courſe there is no remedy but repetition. Thus whoever is indolent is intemperate alſo, and partly from neceſſity ; and the evils neceſſarily following both theſe cauſes often make the rich & great more wretched than the poor, and the ballance of happineſs is held more equally between them ; for however other things may be diſtributed, happineſs, like water, always finds its level among men. I wiſh this obſervation might cure theſe of their envy, and teach the others how to enjoy their wealth.

Before I return to my ſubject, I fear I muſt make an apology for what I am going to ſay, and hope no one will be offended when I venture to ſay that nine in ten of all the chronic diſeaſes in the world, particularly the gout, owe their firſt riſe to intemperance. Many a good man, who piques himſelf upon being the moſt ſober regular creature alive, and never eats but of one or two plain diſhes, as he calls them, nor exceeds his pint of wine at any meal; keeps good hours, and never ſleeps above eight or nine, may be ſurprized, if not affronted, to have his diſeaſe imputed to intemperance ; which he conſiders as a great crime. And yet he is often ill, ſick in his ſtomach, troubled with indigeſtion, and crippled by the gout. The caſe is, we judge of temperance and intemperance from our own habits, without any juft idea of either. What we are ufed to do, and fee others do, we think right, and never go up to nature for our knowledge. The beft way to explain what I mean by intemperance, may be to enquire what is nature's law of temperance, and to deviate from that muft be confidered as intemperance. And here I muft beg leave to obferve, that temperance is a thing of which no Englifhman has or can have the leaft idea, if he judges from his own or his neighbors habits. To form fome notion of it he muft have feen other countries, particularly Spain, Portugal, or Italy, and obferved how men live there. What they call temperance, or even tolerable living, with us would be thought downright ftarving. In this view temperance, is local and comparative ; but what I mean is natural temperance not depending upon place or cuftom (for I do not mean fafting or abftinence, which can never be falutary but after repletion) ; and we muft not judge of it from countries where a piece of bad bread and an onion with a draught of water is thought a tolerable meal ; nor from our own, where beggars live better than the nobles of fome countries, and where we riot in the choice of plenty native and exotic every day.

To come then to my idea of it : I think there is an abfolute, determined temperance, to be meafured by every man's natural unprovoked appetite, digeftion and confumption, while he continues in a good ftate of health, and right habit of life. As long as a man eats and drinks no more than his ftomach calls for, and will bear without the leaft pain, dif-tention, eruĉtation or uneafinefs of any kind; nor than his body confumes and throws off to the laft grain; he may be faid to live in a very prudent well-regulated ftate of temperance, that will probably pre-ferve him in health and fpirits to great old age.

This is nature's law : and the reverfe of it, or in-deed any great deviation from it, muft be intempe-rance. When we eat without appetite, or urged beyond moderate fatiety, provoked by incentives of any kind : when we drink without thirft for the fake of the liquor. Indeed I cannot allow him to be ftriĉtly temperate who drinks any wine or ftrong liquor at all, unlefs it be medicinally, or now and then for the fake of fociety and good humor, but by no means every day.

Now let us compare this fimple idea of temper-rance with the common courfe of moft men's lives, and obferve their progrefs from health to ficknefs : for I fear we fhall find but very few who have any pretenfions to real temperance. In early youth we are infenfibly led into intemperance by the indul-gence and miftaken fondnefs of parents and friends wifhing to make us happy by anticipa-tion. Having thus exhaufted the firft degrees of luxury before we come to the dominion of ourfelves, we fhould find no pleafure in our liberty did we not advance in new fenfations, nor feel our-

E

felves free but as we abufe it. Thus we go on till fome friendly pain or difeafe bids, or rather forces, us to ftop. But in youth all the parts of our bodies are ftrong and flexible, and bear the firft loads of excefs with lefs hurt, and throw them off foon by their own natural vigor and action, or with very little affiftance from artificial evacuations. As we grow older, either by nature in due time, or repeated excefles before our time, the body is lefs able to free itfelf, and wants more aid from art. The man however goes on, taking daily more than he wants, or can poffibly get rid of; he feels himfelf replete and oppreffed, and, his appetite failing, his fpirits fink for want of frefh fupply. He has recourfe to dainties, fauces, pickles, provocatives of all forts. Thefe foon lofe their power; and though he wafhes down each mouthful with a glafs of wine, he can relifh nothing. What is to be done? Send for a phyfician. Doctor, I have loft my ftomach; pray give me, fays he, with great innocence and ignorance, fomething to give me an appetite; as if want of appetite was a difeafe to be cured by art. In vain would the phyfician, moved by particular friendfhip to the man, or that integrity he owes to all men, give him the beft advice in two words, *quære fudando*, feek it by labor. He would be thought a man void of all knowledge and fkill in his profeffion, if he did not immediately, or after a few evacuations, prefcribe ftomachics, bitter fpicy infufions in wine or brandy, vitriolic elixirs, bark, fteel, &c. By the ufe of thefe things the ftomach, roufed to a little extraordinary action, frees itfelf, by difcharging it's crude, auftere, coagulated contents into the bowels, to be thence forwarded into blood. The man is freed for a time, finds he can eat again, and thinks all well. But this is a fhort-liv'd delufion. If he is robuft, the acrimony floating in the blood will be thrown out, and a fit of gout fucceeds ; if lefs fo, rheumatifm or colic, &c. as I have already faid. But let us fuppofe it to be the gout, which if he bears patiently, and lives moderatly, drinking no madeira or brandy to keep it out of his ftomach, nature will relieve him in a certain time and the gouty acrimony concofted and exhaufted by the fymptomatic fever that always attends, he will recover into health ; if affifted by judicious, mild, and foft medicines, his pains might be greatly affuaged and mitigated, and he would recover fooner. But however he recovers, it is but for a fhort time ; for he returns to his former habits, and quickly brings on the fame round of complaints again and again, all aggravated by each return, and he lefs able to bear them ; till he becomes a confirmed invalid and cripple for life, which, with a great deal of ufelefs medication, and a few journies to Bath, he drags on, till, in fpite of all the doftors he has confulted, and the infallible quack medicines he has taken, lamenting that none have been lucky enough to hit his cafe, he finks below opium and brandy, and dies long before his time. This is the courfe I have lived to fee many take, and believe it to be the cafe of more whom I have never heard of, and which any one may obferve in the circle of his acquaintance, all this chain of

evils is brought on and accumulated by indolence
and intemperance, or miftaken choice of diet. How
eafily might they have been remedied, had the real
caufe been known and attended to in time.

I believe I muft here explain a little more fully
what I mean by · provoking the appetite, which I
take to be the general mode of intemperance among
men ; for cuftom has made all kinds of incentives
to excefs fo common, that thofe of daily ufe, far
from being confidered in the clafs of intemperance,
are by moft people thought to be not only falutary
but neceffary ; and they never fufpect the leaft
evil from the common decoraments of the table,
falt, pepper, muftard, vinegar ; and yet, however extraordinary it may feem, I will venture to pronounce
that excefs in any of thefe muft be doubly prejudicial
to health : hurtful in themfelves by their acrimony,
they provoke the appetite beyond natural fatiety to
receive an oppreffive load, which the ftomach it felf
would foon feel, were it not artificially ftimulated
to difcharge it into the blood by wine and ftrong liquors immediately after.   Thus one error brings
on another, and when men have eaten too much,
they drink too much alfo by a kind of neceffity.
He will certainly be a healthier man, who is very
moderate in the ufe of thefe things, than he who exceeds ; they may be fometimes ufeful as medicines ;
but can never add to the wholfomnefs of our daily
food. To give fome weight to what I fay, there are
whole nations in the world that have never known

any of them, and are healthy, ſtrong, and vigorous; I do not mean by this to proſcribe them intirely, eſpecially ſalt and vinegar ; but only to recommend great moderation.

If this be true of the common provocatives at every poor man's board, who is there that exceeds not nature's law ? who is truly temperate ? What ſhall we ſay of that ſtudied, labored, refined extravagance at the tables of the rich, where the culinary arts are puſhed to that exceſs, that luxury is become falſe to itſelf, and things are valued, not as they are good and agreeable to the natural and undebauched appetite ; but high, inflammatory, rare, out of ſeaſon, and coſtly ; where, though variety is aimed at, every thing has the ſame taſte, and nothing it's own. I am ſorry and aſhamed, that men profeſſing luxury ſhould underſtand it ſo little, as to think it lies in the diſh or the ſauce or multitude of either ; or that urging beyond natural ſatiety can afford any real enjoyment. But this they do by all the reſearches of culinary and medical art, introducing all the foreign aids to luxury, every ſtimulating provocative that can be found in acids, ſalts, fiery ſpices, and eſſences of all kinds, to rouſe their nerves to a little feeling ; not knowing the more they are chafed and irritated the more callous they ſtill grow ; and the ſame things muſt now be more frequently repeated, increaſed in quantity, and exalted in quality, till they know not where to ſtop, and every meal they make ſerves only to overload and oppreſs the ſtomach, to foul and inflame the blood, obftruct and choak all the capillary channels, bring on a hectic fever of irritation, that though it raife the fpirits for the evening, leaves behind it all the horrid fenfations of inanition and crapula the next morning; and but that nature is fo kind as to ftop them in their career with a painful fit of gout or fome other illnefs, in which fhe gets a little refpite, they would foon be at the end of their courfe.

Men bring all thefe evils upon themfelves, either not knowing or not attending to two things: the one, that pleafure is a coy coquet, and to be enjoyed muft not always be purfued; we muft fometimes fit ftill, that fhe may come and court us in her turn: the other, that pleafure and happinefs are as diftinct things as riot and enjoyment: befides, pleafure is not infinite, and our fenfations are limited: we can bear but a certain meafure, and all urging beyond it, infallibly brings pain in it's ftead. Let the men of high experience bear me teftimony, that this is true of all the luxuries of the table, wine, mufic, women, and every fenfuality.

Thefe men may tell me, perhaps that I have made a mighty fine declamation againft luxury and intemperance: but what is this to the purpofe? they defire not to be told of their faults, nor to hear dif-agreeable truths which they know already. Have I no art or fkill to reconcile health and luxury, no remedy, no rare fecret to repair and reftore fenfa-tion and vigour worn to rags? No Medea's kettle.

to boil anew ? If not, do not defcribe to us a life of moderation, temperance, and exercife : it is not worth having upon thefe terms. I am aware of the unreafonable expectations of many, that their demands would rife high, fome of them to the impoffible. At prefent I am only fetting forth the caufes ; when I come to talk of remedy, I will endeavour to convince them that the artificial helps they expect are not in nature, but that there are in nature ways and means by which many gouty, broken conftitutions, that have been defpaired of, might be repaired and reftored to a very defirable degree of health and enjoyment. But I muft firft fay a word or two to the intemperate or miftaken in the middle clafs of life.

In England all degrees of men are furnifhed with the means of intemperance, and therefore it is no wonder that moft men are intemperate. If they are lefs fo in other countries, it is not that they have more virtue, but they want the means : their oppreffive governments, the precarious ftate of property, and their fuperftitious religion, keep them fo poor that luxury is not in their power. They have however this advantage from their poverty, that they are much lefs afflicted with chronic difeafes than we are. I verily believe there are more gouts in England, than in all the reft of Europe : a proof that good living is more univerfal. But not to the advocates for this good living do I wifh to addrefs myfelf ; I fear they will be as incorrigible as their fuperiors in higher and more refined luxury. But there are fome not intemperate from choice, but example, habit, cuftom,

miftake, not knowing their daily diet to be unwholfome, and productive of their difeafes. To thefe it
may be of fome ufe to have the unwholfome pointed
out, and their choice directed to better things. Men
of laborious occupations, who work in the open air,
can and do bear great exceffes and much unwholfome diet without much hurt : I never knew a fick
or gouty gardener that was not a remarkable fot.
But men of fedentary trades and bufinefs, fhop-
keepers of all kinds, feel much fooner and more
heavily the ill effects of intemperence or miftaken
choice in their meat and drink. Their firft care
therefore ought to be, not to add the difeafes of intemperance to thofe of inactivity, but proportion
what they take, as well in quantity, as in quality,
to their confumption. But let us fee how well they do
this. They all fay they live upon plain things, and
never indulge in made difhes ; but they will eat hear-
tily of a goofe or duck, with a large quantity of fage,
onion, pepper and falt, a pig with fimilar preparation, and a hare with higher and more compounded
feafoning. Do they ever eat veal without ftuffing,
or even a leg of mutton without caper-fauce ?
If ever they eat a fteak or a chop, if it is fometimes
without pepper, I believe it is never without
pickles, the worft of all poifons. They are furprized that fuch meals fhould rife on their ftomachs with flatulence, four and bitter hiccups and
eructations, which, if they did not keep them down
with a fufficient quantity of wine or fometimes a
dram, they would be troubled with all the time of
digeftion. If this method fucceeds fo far as to quiet
their ftomachs for the prefent, they go on with it,

regardlefs or ignorant of future and diftant confequences. Thus are thefe fharp, harfh, hot and inflammatory things forced out of the ftomach into
the blood, before it has had time to dilute and fubdue, or reject them, and the fuperfluous load they
bring along with them. And thus is laid the foundation of every difeafe, that appears when thefe acrid
and fiery particles are accumulated in the blood to
a certain degree,

There are others whofe pretenfions to plain diet
may feem better founded, but who neverthelefs eat,
and are fond of, things unwholfome, and very un-
fit for men of fedentary lives; fuch as falted and
fmoaked flefh and fifh of all kinds, hams, tongues,
heavy flour puddings, toafted cheefe, &c. all which
are of fuch hard and indiffoluble texture, that they
never diffolve well in the ftomach of a plowman :
the fame falt, feafoning, and fmoke which harden
and preferve them from putrefaction before they are
eaten, keep them from diffolution afterwards, fo
that they never are digefted at all ; nor is it poffible
any good nourifhment fhould ever come from them :
the falts they contain are indeed melted in the in-
teftinal juices, and get into the blood, producing,
in the beft conftitutions, thofe tettery, itchy, or
fcaly eruptions, commonly but very erroneoufly
called the fcurvy, which is quite another kind of
difeafe. To this kind of food is owing the bad
health of country people, and their children's rick-
ety heads and limbs, and big and hard bellies.

F

Another capital miftake many people fall into, who in other refpects are very moderate in their diet, is, that the flefh-meat they eat is always over-done ; if boiled too much, the juices are loft ; if over-roafted fried, or broiled, the action of the fire continued too long, changes the mild animal flefh into fomething of another quality ; the fat is made bitter and rancid, which fire will always do by the fweeteft oil ; and the fcorched outfide of the lean, dry and acrimonious : the lefs therefore all flefh-meat undergoes the power of fire, the milder and wholfomer it is. I do not mean by this to recommend the cuftoms of Cannibals and Tartars who eat raw flefh ; or beafts of prey, that devour animals a-live : but it may be obferved, that the firft are free from our difeafes, and the others amazingly ftrong & vigorous. We may learn this from them at leaft, that our meat cannot be the wholefomer for being, as fome call it, thoroughly done ; and that we fhould learn to like it with fome of its red juices unfpoiled by the fire. Upon this principle the Englifh cookery is to be perferred to the French, who ftew and roaft to rags ; and of Englifh cookery broiling muft be the beft.

This leads me to another obfervation, which perhaps none but phyficans, or thofe who have ftudied well the nature of man and his aliments, are able to make. It is this : that man being born to devour moft of the fruits and animals of the earth and water, there ought to be a certain proportion of animal and vegetable ftubftances in his food ; the animal tending fpontaneoufly to putrefaction; the vegetable correcting that tendency from going too far : thus from the due mixture of both qualities refults that neutral proprety, equally diftant from acid as alkali, that is effentially neceffary to produce good blood. This is fo manifeft, that who ever will obferve attentively may fee, whenever either of thefe prevails in body, there is fo ftrong a defire and longing for things of the other fort, as well as pleafing fenfation in the palate and ftomach when they are taken, as plainly indicate the natural want. Let a man have lived long upon flefh-meat wholly, he will have a moft eager appetite for fruit and vegetables ; and if kept too long without them, as is the cafe with thofe who have lived fome time at fea, will grow fick of the real fcurvy ; but if before they are too far gone they reach the land, they will eat the firft common grafs they can come at, with more avidity than a horfe or ox, and be perfectly cured by it. In like manner they who have lived long upon vegetables (which regimen is often prefcribed to invalids, efpecially in the gout) will have great craving for flefh-meat. We ought to learn from all this to attend diligently to the calls of nature, and ballance the mixture with due proportion, not only that our vitals may have the lefs labor in preparing and making our juicies fit for nourifhment, but to prevent the difeafes that are peculiar to the predominancy of either. And here I may obferve, that the error of moft men's diet in every clafs of life is, that the acid, crude and auftere, almoft always abound : not that they do not eat flefh-meat enough, but they fpoil it in the preparation and cookery, changing its animal nature

into fomething worfe than vegetable, taking off in.
tirely all its tendency to diffolution and putrefaction
by falting, fmoking, pickling, potting, and preferv-
ing things that in their own fimple nature would
foon corrupt and diffolve ; but by thefe preparations
are hardened and embalmed to keep for years like
mummies. The fame may be faid of every
kind of made difhes ; the falts, fpices, hot
herbs and acids, with which they are feafoned
and compounded, preferve and harden them to
keep for ever : the fauces and gravies they fwim
in have the fame effect as fo much pickle. The
things we feed upon ought all to be in a perifhable
ftate, or they will never furnifh the materials of good
blood ; and what ever is hardned or feafoned fo as
to keep long before it be eaten ought not be eaten
at all, for it will never diffolve in the ftomach.

The nature of moft chronic difeafes, and their firft
fymptom heartburn, as it is commonly called, plainly
fhew the original caufe to be acid crudity prevailing in
the juices ; producing coagulations, concretions and
obftructions of various kinds ; all which are very
manifeft in the gout, rheumatifm, ftone, and moft
nervous cafes : the remedies alfo, that fometimes relieve and palliate, confirm this ; fuch as the volatile al-
kalies, hartfhorn, falt ammoniac, teftaceous powders,
fope, &c. Many may be furprized at this, and fay,
it cannot be ; for, though they have thefe difeafes,
they take little or no acids : but there are many things
they take that are acefcent, that is liable to become

acid, efpecially by the heat of the ftomach. This they are not aware of; but they are in their nature much more prejudicial than things already four: for, befides that people take not thefe in any quantity, the acefcent never become four but by the act of fermentation, which, being raifed in the ftomach where it ought never to happen, produces ftrange tumults, wind, vapor, gas, that is, that fume arifing from fermenting liquors of any kind, which has been known fometimes to kill at a ftroke. It may here be neceffary to enumerate fome of thofe things called acefcent. Thefe are fweets of every kind, puddings, cakes, paftry, creams, confections, &c. and every thing made of flour, efpecially fermented; bread in particular, fo far from being the wholfome thing many imagine, is not only unholfome by its acefcency, but, by the ftrong ferment it contains, whenever it predominates, it forces into fermentation every thing capable of it, that it meets with in the ftomach * : the bread of London I fear is particularly fo; partly by being robbed of its bran, which in fome degree would foften and correct it, but chiefly by having in it, befides its ufual ferment, a great quantity of four alum, moft abfurdly added to make it unnaturally white.† Many eat bread from principle, and like it by habit; take a flice between meals, and

* Whoever requires proof of this, may have it by the following experiment: Put a common toaft into half a pint of water, and let it ftand fix or eight hours near the fire, fo as to be kept in the heat of the human ftomach, and it will be four as vinegar.

† To be convinced of this, boil a pound of common London bread in a fufficient quantity of water to make it

with their fruit as a corrector ; and think a bit of
bread and glafs of wine a moft abftemious excellent
fupper. I think they are miftaken in all this, and
that bread ought to be eaten but fparingly, and for
want of other and better vegetables. In this light
we muft alfo confider moft forts of feafonings, ftuffing, force-meats, and compounded fauces. But the
greateft acefcent, or rather bane of all, high and low,
rich or otherwife, whoever they are that take it conftantly, is wine : wine alone produces more difeafes
than all the other caufes put together. All men
allow that wine taken to excefs is hurtful : they fee
the immediate evils that follow ; but diftant effects,
that require more attentive and deducive obfervation,
very few fee or believe ; and judging from prefent
and agreeable feelings, they fay that a little wine is
wholfome, and good for every one, and accordingly
take it every day, give it their children, and teach
them to like it by debauching their natural tafte in
the earlieft infancy : thus they come to relifh it by
habit, and to be uneafy without it, like fnuff takers
without their tobacco : the want is equally habitual
and unnatural in both cafes ; for the ftomach wants
wine no more than the nofe does fnuff : the immediate fenfation of both, after a little ufe, is pleafant ; but
the remote effect of wine taken conftantly infinitely
more pernicious than of the fnuff. This hurts the
nofe only ; the other accumulating a little indigeftion

thick as gruel. Let it ftand to fubfide ; pour off the clear,
and boil away all the water ; the alum will be found at
bottom, mixed with a little common falt.

every day, corrupts all the juices of the body moft effentially. And though it be often taken with a view to promote digeftion and affift the operations of the ftomach, it manifeftly does harm to both. Inftead of digefting and diffolving, it hardens, and prevents diffolution, and curdles and corrupts the milky chyle and firft juices produced from our food. It warms indeed and ftimulates the ftomach to greater exertion than is natural or neceffary, and thereby enables it to difcharge it's contents the fooner; whence that agreeable feel of warmth and comfort from it's immediate action. But by this extraordinary action it forces our food out of the ftomach too foon, before it is foftened, diffolved, and properly prepared, and fends it into the bowels crude, hard, and auftere, in that ftate to be carried into the blood, there to produce every kind of difeafe. Whatever therefore the advocates for a little wine every day may think, or argue in favor of it ; they are moft undoubtedly in a very great error, and it were certainly much better and fafer to drink a bottle and get a little merry once a week, drinking water only or fmall beer at all other times : in which interval nature might totally fubdue it, and recover intirely. Water is the only liquor nature knows of or has provided for all animals ; and whatever nature gives us, we may depend upon it, is fafeft and beft for us. Accordingly we fee that when we have committed any exceffes or miftakes of any kind, and fuffer from them, it is water that relieves. Hence the chief good of Bath, Spa, and many other medicinal waters, efpecially to hard drinkers. It is the element that dilutes and carries off crudities and indigeſtions, &c. the mineral virtues they contain may make them tolerable to the ſtomach in their paſſage, but do, as I believe, little more in the body : it is the water that cures.   Wine, if it be not of our own inventions, was given us as a cordial in ſickneſs, wearineſs, ſorrow, and old age, and a moſt ſalutary charm it would be for moſt of theſe evils, did we not exhauſt it's power by daily uſe, and inſtead of taking it as ſuch, drink it up as common draught in youth and health to make us mad. I know this is a very tender topic to touch upon, and too favorite a pleaſure to argue againſt, with any reaſonable hope of convincing ; moſt men having ſo indulged themſelves in this bewitching habit, that they think they cannot live without a little wine every day, & their very exiſtence depends upon it ; their ſtomachs require it, nature calls for it, St. Paul adviſes it, it muſt be good. Thus men catch at every ſhadow of an argument that favors their inclinations.   St. Paul adviſes it as a medicine ſometimes, but certainly not every day. There is no medicine I know of, that, taken every day, will not either ceaſe to act entirely, or by acting too much do harm.   It will be ſaid, that many drink wine every day without gout, ſtone, or any diſeaſe at all in conſequence of it.   I believe not many, or I ſhould know ſome of them. If any are ſo ſtrong as to bear it to old age unhurt, they muſt be very active as well as ſtrong to ſubdue it. But I have nothing to ſay to theſe ; my buſineſs is with invalids who complain, and certainly ought not to meaſure conſtitutions with thoſe above their match. The same arguments will hold equally in favor of every other bad habit. Your nose will want it's snuff, your palate it's spices ; and when the fashion was for women to be small waisted, their galled sides grown callous by the long compression of the stays wanted their support. Nature, like a true female, cries out at the first violence, but submits in time, is reconciled, and grows fond of the ravisher. But it is the business of philosophers to distingush carefully between the real wants of nature and the artificial calls of habit ; and when we find these begin to hurt us, we ought to make the utmost persevering efforts to break the enchantment of bad customs ; and though it cost us some uneasy sensations at first, we must bear them patiently ; they will not kill ; and a very little time will reconcile us to better modes of life.

There is another capital mistake many labor under in the choice of their wine, preferring the strong, hot, and coarse sorts, Medeira, Port, Mountain, &c. to the milder, more elegant, and certainly less unwholsome French and Italian wines, accounting them better for the stomach, and good against wind, &c. My observation has been, that they who use these strong stomach wines to cure wind are never free from it, and all the gouty disorders of indigestion. Indeed, it cannot well be otherwise ; for there is nothing so repugnant to natural digestion as the use of these strong liquors, which instead of dissolving hard-

en every thing ; and thus for ever, when the firſt
warmth is gone off, leave a crapulary, crude, four
load of yeſterday, to ferment, fret, and irritate the
ſtomach and bowels every day.

Thus have I endeavored to point out two of the
true primary, capital cauſes of the gout, and moſt
other chronic diſeaſes ; and moſt ſincerely wiſh that
what 1 have ſaid may engage thoſe whom it moſtly
concerns, the gouty, the infirm and valetudinary of
every claſs, to obſerve, reflect, and think for themſelves upon the hints 1 have thrown out ; in which
light what I have ſaid, muſt be conſidered, rather
than as logical or demonſtrative proof. I know the
reaſoning and arguments may be much improved
and carried farther, and if I had more leiſure I might
have attempted it : but I am well aware of the un-
ſurmountable difficulty of convincing men againſt
their will by any arguments at all. I chuſe therefore at preſent to invite them to ſelf-conviction from
there own obſervations and experience. I flatter
myſelf they will find it well worth their pains, to
reaſon a little more than they do with and for themſelves ; and it will be a great point gained for them,
if it turn their miſled opinions from all that imaginary power of reſtoring health in any of that multitude of ridiculous and moſt truly contemptible medicines, that are daily obtruded upon the public,
with endleſs lies to recommend them, by a ſet of the
pooreſt, moſt ignorant and paltry rogues in the na-
tion ; and engage their attention to their true reme-

dy, a right inftitution of life. In judging of which, if they find themfelves unequal to the tafk, they may be affifted by men of humanity, fkill, and honefty.

Of VEXATION.

I COME now to the laft general caufe of chronic difeafes, Vexation. A very fruitful parent of many bodily evils, producing generally difeafes of inanition, much more difficult, not only to be cured, but relieved, than thofe we fuffer either from Indolence or Intemperance. But as it is not fo common a caufe of the gout as the other two, it may not be neceffary to confider it very minutely at prefent. I fhall not therefore enter deeply into the regions of metaphyfical conjecture, nor run wild after my own conceits, or theirs who have gone aftray before me, in gueffing at the incomprehenfible union of foul and body, and their mutual powers of acting upon each other. I fhall content myfelf with obferving only, what may be of fome ufe, that every great degree of vexation, whether in the fhape of anger, envy, refentment, difcontent or forrow, has moft deftructive and deleterious effects upon the vitals of the body, whether fudden and violent, or flow and lafting.

The firft immediate effect of violent grief or vexation is to take off the action of the ftomach intirely.

Let us suppofe a man, in the beft health, the higheft good humor and fpirits, as well as good ftomach, fitting down to dinner with his friends, receives fuddenly fome very afflicting news. Inftantly his appetite is gone, and he can neither eat nor fwallow a morfel. Let the fame thing happen after he has made a hearty, chearful meal, as fuddenly the action of his ftomach, the whole power of digeftion is cut off totally, as if it were become paralytic ; and what he has eaten lies a moft oppreffive load. Prehaps, as the excefs of weaknefs is often convulfion, it may be rejected by a violent vomit, or do greater mifchief. For which reafon fuch ftrokes of diftrefs are lefs hurtful received upon an empty than a full ftomach. But why is this ? what connexion is there between a piece of bad news and a mans ftomach full or empty ? Whatever the caufe be, the effect is certain and invariable. Is it becaufe the animal fpirits, or the action of the nerves, whatever be the fecret caufe of their power, is called of to fupply and fupport the tumultuous agitation of the brain, and the ftomach, with all it's appendages and their fecretions, is left powerlefs and paralytic, and muft therefore either act convulfively or not at all ?

Befides this pernicious effect of perverting the natural action of the ftomach and inteftines, the whole circulation of the blood is difturbed. The contraction and dilatation of the heart, that is,the alternate action by which it opens to receive the blood from the veins, and clofes again to force it out through the arteries; which operation ought to be as true and certain as the vibrations of a pendulum; are broken and uneven: the heart flutters, palpitates; now is overloaded with blood and in danger of suffocation, now receives none at all: consequently all the secretions muft be as irregular, some of the glands receiving too abundant a supply, that either hurries through, or oppreffes and overpowers them, others none at all. Hence that hafty gufhing of pale limpid urine in amazing quantities, thofe fudden burfts of unmeaning tears: fometimes great drynefs and choaking thirft, fometimes the overflowing of the mouth with water inftead of faliva, and many other nervous and hyfterical affections, fits, fyncope, epilepfy, &c. all which indicate the greateft tumults and perturbations in the inmoft receffes of the nervous and vital frame. Many kinds of difeafe have fprung from this fountain, of fuch unaccountably horrid and terrifying appearances, that formerly they could no otherwife account for them, but by the malefice of forcery, and the immediate poffeffion of devils.

In fhort, more filent, but longer continued grief, the effects are fimilar, but not fo violent. Many little ftrokes repeated will do the fame thing in time that a great blow does at once. The function of the ftomach will be more gently difturbed and perverted, it's juices vitiated, and all it's contents will forever turn four, bitter, or rancid; fo that no mild milky chyle, or wholfome material of nourifhment, can ever come into the blood. The patient muft languish with cachectic inanition, univerſal bad habit of body, or pine and waſte with atrophy, the want of nouriſhing ſupply ; whence ariſe complications of various diſeaſes ſucceeding each other, always from bad to worſe : and unleſs he can ſubdue his anxiety, and reſtore peace of mind, he muſt in time ſink under it, and die, as it is ſaid, of a broken heart.

Whoever vexes long, muſt certainly want nouriſhment ; for, beſides the diſturbed ſtate of the ſtomach, it's broken appetite and bad digeſtion, from whence what ſupply there is muſt come not only ill prepared, but vitiated, into the blood ; there can be no ſleep in this ſtate of mind : the perturbed ſpirit cannot reſt ; and it is in ſleep that all nouriſhment is preformed, and the finer parts of the body, chafed and worn with the fatigue of the day, are repaired and reſtored to their natural vigor. While we are awake this cannot ſo well be done ; becauſe the inceſſant action of the body or mind, being always partial and irregular, prevents that equal diſtribution of the blood to all parts alike, from which each fibre and filament receives that ſhare or portion that ſuits it beſt. In ſleep, when it is quiet and natural, all the muſcles of the body, that is, all its active powers that are ſubject to our will, are lulled to reſt, compoſed and relaxed into a genial, temporary kind of palſy, that leaves not the leaſt obſtruction or hindrance of the paſſage of the blood to every atom. Accordingly the pulſe is always ſlower and more equal, the reſpiration deeper and more regular, and the ſame degree of vital warmth diffuſed a-

like through every part ; fo that the extremities are
equally warm with the heart.

Vexation operating in this manner upon the or-
gans of digeition and concoction, and difturbing
and obftructing the natural progrefs of nutrition,
mult often produce difeafes fimiliar to thofe of long-
continued intemperance ; it's firft effect being indigeftion with all it's fymptoms, wind, eructation,
heart-burn, hiccup, &c. It is no wonder therefore
it fhould fometimes bring on a fit of gout, which as
I have faid, is manifeftly a difeafe of crudity and indigeftion ; and often the gout in the flomach and
bowels. Indeed moft cold crude colics are of this
kind. Schirrous concretions will alfo be formed in
the fpleen, liver, glands of the mefentery, and
throughout the whole fyftem of the belly. Many of
thefe indurated tumors will appear outwardly, fo as
to be felt by the hand ; thefe in time will degenerate into cancers and cancerous ulcerations, and
many fatal evils, not the leaft of which, in my opinion, is, that the patient will fuffer a long time before he dies.

All the paffions, when they are inordinate, may
have injurious effects upon the vital frame : exceffive joy has fometimes given a fatal blow, and fudden burfts of laughter done great mifchiefs, efpecially to delicate or weakly people who have often been
thrown into fpafms, cramps, convulfions, hyfteric fits
and hæmorrhages by them. But as I think the

word Vexation comprehends the chief of thofe paffions that hurt us moft,and mean not to make a me.
taphyfical enquiry about them, it is needlefs to be
particular upon each. It may fuffice to have fhewn
the immediate and remote influence of vexation upon the human body.

Whatever men may think of their difeafes, their
ftrange fymptoms & appearances, and their unaccoun-
table caufes, thefe are the three original great fources
of moft of the chronic difeafes of mankind ; which
I have endeavored to fet forth and explain in fo fa-
miliar a manner, that I hope I have been perfectly
intelligible to every one who will venture to think
and judge for himfelf. To fuch rational people only
ly I addrefs myfelf ; and to enable them to do this
the better, I have furnifhed thefe hints and obfervations, which may be extended, improved and applied to particular cafes. I want not, nor wifh to
obtrude my ideas upon any man, however warranted
I may think myfelf from the obfervation and experience of my whole life : my principal aim has been
only to make men ftop a little in their career, and
confider with themfelves whether it may not be poffible for them to be miftaken, even in that courfe
of diet and thofe habits of life which they never fuf-
pected. If they are ill, and for any time, there
muft be a more fubftantial caufe for it, than they
are in general willing to allow. It is not always
catching cold, for we do not catch cold fo often as
we think we do ; and when a healthy robuft perfon
takes cold, which can happen but rarely, if this be

the whole of the difeafe, it cannot laft long. But the truth is, when the crudity, fuperfluity and acrimony of an indolent, intemperate life have accumulated to fuch a degree as to make us fick, then we fay we have taken cold, or complain of a bad conftitution, when we have fpoiled perhaps a very good one; or with Sydenham, that the epidemic conftitution of the air has infected us, or that this or that trifle has difagreed. I am fully and firmly perfuaded, that whoever will reflect with fome degree of intelligence and fanity, be juft to himfelf, and candid with his phyfician, will in general be able to trace his complaints and difeafes up to one or other of thefe three caufes. And whoever does this, muft infallibly fee how vain and idle all his hopes and expectations of lafting remedy and eftablifhed health muft be from any kind of quack medicines, or indeed the common and too general practice of phyfic, when the whole is refted upon fomething given to fwallow; how inadequate the means are to the end propofed and hoped for; how ill vomiting and purging can fupply the place of temperance; bleeding, bliftering, and all artificial evacuation, of activity; cordials & opium, of peace of mind. Is not this to fill the body with harfh & unholfome juices, and then tear it to pieces to get them out again? To make artificial holes and fores in the fkin to renew the blood and difcharge fuperfluities, inftead of employing mufcular motion to rub off and grind down all the acrimony of angular aculeated particles, and make them fmooth and round, & eafily divifible; and to employ

11

intoxication and ftupefaction to take off the fenfe of pain, and leave the caufe where it was, or fix it faftter ? Can any reafonable perfon hope for health or long life by any of thefe unnatural methods, when thefe only are employed ? Let him look round among his neighbours and acquaintance, and tell me whether, n&c only all the gouty, but rheumatic, colicky, jaundiced, paralytic, dropfical, hyfterical people he has ever feen, are not either always fo, or by fits fo; and whether thofe returning paroxyfms or fits of thefe diforders do not always grow worfe and worfe, in fpite of all their medication and quackery, till a complication or apoplexy comes on, that at laft, though long before their time, puts an end to their miferable lives. Thefe evils are confidered as the inheritance of human nature,unavoidable & incurable, and fubmitted to in abfolute defpair ; though there has not one rational attempt, that I know of, ever yet been made to remedy them in earneft. All the methods hitherto employed have only been to relieve, and thofe often fo pernicioufly, that the future health has been facrificed to obtain prefent relief or eafe. This muft for ever be the cafe when in chronic cafes it is obtained by art, and nature has no fhare : or where the phyfician does all, and the patient nothing for himfelf.

Of the Cure of the Gout and all other Chronic Diſeaſes, and the Repair of a brokenConſtitution.

HAVING ſet forth the real caufes of the gout, & all it's congenial diſeaſes, I come now to the moſt eſſential part, to adminſter all poſſible comfort to thoſe whom great pain and long ſuffering may have made attentive and docile, and willing to take health upon the terms it is poſſible to have it. To the young and voluptuous, who are yet in their career, and declare for a ſhort life and a merry one, I have nothing to ſay but this, that a ſhort life is very ſeldom a merry one; on the contrary, is generally made up of a few years of riotous pleaſure without happineſs, to be ſeverely paid for by as many more of pain, ſickneſs, regret and deſpair.

Having ſhewn that the gout is not hereditary, not inherent in our conſtitutions, but produced by the daily accumulations of indigeſted, unſubdued acrimony and ſuperfluity, which, when they abound to a certain degree, muſt end either in a fit of the gout or ſome other diſeaſe, according to the conſtitution, as long as any vigor is left in the body; for nature will for ever free or endeavour to free itſelf, and purge the blood of its impurities by gout, by fever, by pain of one kind or other, that takes off the appetite, and for a time gives reſpite, and prevents the pouring in of more and more enemies to diſturb it's operation, and make it ineffectual. Thus young people, after a fit of gout is happily and well gone off, are as free from it as if they had never had it; and if they would take warning and be careful not to breed it again, moſt certainly would for ever remain free. How abſurd therefore, how ridiculouſly igno-rant muſt be every attempt to cure the gout *in futuro* by medicine, before it be yet formed, before it has any exiſtence !   Can ſuch a medicine give ſuperna-tural ſtrength, and enable an old man living ſin in-dolence to digeſt and conſume, or diſcharge the ſu-perfluities of his daily intemperance ? that is, to give him more vigorous powers than nature gave him at one-and-twenty, or when the gout came firſt upon him.   The Duke of Portland's powder promiſed to do ſomething like this, and moſt certainly kept off the gout for two or three years.   But what was it ? and what did it really do ?   It was a ſtrong ſpicy bitter taken in ſubſtance, in a large quantity, for a long time ; its effect was to keep up a conſtant fe-ver as long as it was taken ; this kept the gouty matter always afloat, and prevented its fixing any where.   But there was no living long with a conſtant fever ; accordingly many of thoſe who took it died very ſoon.   I myſelf obſerved between fifty and ſixty of it's advocates, ſome my patients, ſome my acquaintance or neighbors, who were apparently cured by it for a little while ; but in leſs than ſix years time, *omnes ad internecionem cæſi,* they all died to a man.

Many similar attempts have been made with other medicines to cure not only the gout, but moſt other chronic diſeaſes, and with the ſame fatal effects. Antimony and Mercury elaborated into poiſons by chemiſtry have been adminiſtered, particularly the ſolution of ſublimate has torn many a ſtomach to rags, ſo that it could never bear common food afterwards. The deadly night-ſhade, and hemlock, and many ſuch dreadful poiſons, have been given as alteratives to reſtore health. The intention here ſeems to be, kill or cure, to raiſe a violent · agitation or fever in the body, in hopes it may prove ſtrong enough to throw off the diſeaſe and medicine together. The effect has ever been, notwithſtanding a little apparent and deceitful relief may have been perceived from the firſt efforts, that it has ſunk under both loads, and, exhauſted by repeated ſtraining, much ſooner than by the diſeaſe alone.

Can any one in his ſenſes ſuppoſe that diſeaſes a man has been his whole life contracting, and to which he is adding every day by perſeverance in unwholeſome diet, and bad habits, are to be thus removed by a *coup de main ou de baguette ?* or that they will not return, be they cured or conjured away ever ſo often, whilſt he continues the ſame mode of life that brought them on at firſt ?

What then is to be done ? how and in what manner are chronic diſeaſes and cachexies to be cured, and health reſtored and eſtabliſhed ? I have already ſhewn that the cauſes of theſe evils are Indolence, Intemperance, and Vexation; and if there be any truth or weight in what I have ſaid, the remedies are obvious: Activity, Temperance, and Peace of Mind. It will be ſaid the remedies are obvious, but impracticable. Would you bid the feeble cripple, who cannot ſtand, take up his bed and walk ? the man who has loſt all appetite, abſtain ? and the ſleepleſs wretch racked with pain enjoy peace of mind ? No certainly; I am not ſo abſurd. Theſe muſt be aſſiſted by medicine; and if they have not exhauſted all it's power already, a little reſpite, a favourable interval may be obtained, that, with o-ther artificial aids co-operating, may be greatly im-proved to their advantage, and if rightly employed they may get on from ſtrength to ſtrength, till they recover into perfect health. But it is not my de-ſign at preſent to expatiate upon that particular kind of medical relief which every chronic caſe may re-quire; it would lead me into too wide a field, and too far from my preſent purpoſe, which is to ſhew that the gout, in moſt of its ſtages and degrees, may be cured, a preſent paroxyſm or fit relieved, it's re-turn for ever ſafely prevented, and the patient eſta-bliſhed in perfect health.

Let us ſuppoſe the caſe of a man from forty to fifty years of age, who has had at leaſt twenty fits of gout; by which moſt of his joints have been ſo clogged, & obſtructed, as to make walking or any kind of motion very uneaſy to him; let him have had it ſometimes in his ftomach, a little in his head, and often all over him, fo as to make him univerfally fick and low-fpirited, efpecially before a regular fit has come to relieve him. This I apprehend to be as bad a cafe as we need propofe, and that it will not be expected that every old cripple whofe joints are burnt to chalk, and his bones grown together and united by anchy-lofis, who muft be carried from his bed to his table and back again, fhould be propofed as an object of medication and cure; and yet even he might per-haps receive fome relief and palliation in pain, if he has any great degree of it, which is not very com-mon in this cafe. Let us therefore fuppofe the firft example.

If the point be to affuage the violent raging of a prefent paroxyfm; this may be fafely done by giv-ing fome foft and flowly-operating laxative, neither hot nor cold, but warm, either in fmall dofes repeat-ed fo as to move the patient once or twice in twen-ty-four hours, or by a larger dofe oftener in lefs time, according to the ftrength and exigency. This may be followed by a few lenient abforbent correc-tors of acrimony or even gentle anodynes : proper cataplafms may alfo be fafely applied to the raging part, which often affuage pain furprizingly; with as much mild and fpontaneoufly-diffolving nourifh-ment as may keep the fpirits from finking too low : but I would wifh them to fink a little, and exhort the patient to bear that lownefs with patience and refignation, till nature, affifted by foft and fucculent food, can have time to relieve him. This eafy method of treating a fit of the gout would anfwer in any age ; and if the patient was young and vigorous, and the· pain violent, there could be no danger in taking away a little blood. Thus in two or three days time I have often feen a fevere fit mitigated and made tolerable : and this is a better · way of treating it with regard to future confequences, than bearing it with patience and fuffering it to take i. s courfe : for the fooner the joints are relieved from diftenfion and pain, the lefs danger there is of obftru6tions fixing in them, or their being calcined and utterly deftroyed. But inftead of this, the general pra6tice is quite the reverfe. Oh ! keep up your fpirits, they cry ; keep it out of your ftomach at all events ; where, whenever it rages in a diftant part, it is not at all inclined to come. As you cannot eat, you muft drink the more freely. So they take cordials, ftrong wines, and rich fpoon-meats. By urging in this manner, a great fever is raifed, the pain enraged and prolonged ; and a fit, that would have ended fpontaneoufly in lefs than a week, protra6ted to a month or fix weeks, and, when it goes off at laft, leaves fuch obftru6tion and weaknefs in the parts, as cripple the man ever after. All this I hope will be fairly and candidly underftood ; for there is doubtlefs a great variety of gouty cafes, but no cafe that will not admit of medical affiftance judicioufly adminiftered.

But the moft capital point of all, and what is moftly defired by all, is to prevent it's return, or changing into any other difeafe, and to eftablifh health. Moft men would be very well pleafed and happy could this be done by any medical trick or noftrum, with full liberty of living as they lift, and indulg· ing every appetite and paffion without controul. Some poor filly creatures, ignorant of all philofophy and the nature of caufes and effects, have been led into experiments of this kind by a few artful rogues, v. 'y much to the prejudice of their future health, and danger of their lives alfo ; expecting from medicine, what it never did or can perform alone, the cure of chronic difeafes.

I think it needlefs here to take any pains to fhew the inefficacy of all the common modes of practice, vomiting, purging, bleeding, bliftering, iffues, &c. They have been found ineffectual not only in the gout, but all other chronic cafes. All fenfible practitioners muft know their effects to be but temporary, & that they are meant and ufed only as means of prefent relief. Let us fee therefore by what practicable plan or regimen the perfon here difcribed, when a fit of the gout is happily ended, may for ever prevent it's return, and fo confirm his general health that it fhall not again be overfet by every flight cold or trifling accident.

I have already fhewn that a certain degree of activity or bodily motion is neceffary at intervals every day, to raife the circulation to that pitch, that

I

will keep the fine veſſels open and the old blood pure, and alſo make new from the freſh juices. If the patient cannot be brought to this, he has no chance of recovering to perfect health. If therefore he can neither walk nor ride at all, he muſt by de-gees be brought to do both by the aſſiſtance of o-thers, which may be given him in the following man. ner: Let a handy active ſervant or two be employ-ed to rub him all over, as he lies in bed, with flan-nels, or flannel gloves, fumigated with gums and ſpices, which will contribute greatly to brace and ſtrenghten his nerves and fibres, and move his blood without any fatigue to himſelf *. This may take up from five to ten minutes at firſt, but muſt be repeated five or ſix times a day, ſuppoſing him to-tally unable to help himſelf. But if he can walk a hundred yards only, it will forward him greatly to walk thoſe hundred yards every two hours, and if he can bear a carriage, let him go out in it every day, till he begins to be tired. The firſt day or two all this may diſturb and fatigue him a little; but if he has patience to perſevere to the fourth, I

* This may ſeem but a trifling preſcription to thoſe who have never tried it ſuſficiently, but is of the utmoſt conſe-quence, and it's effects are amazing; eſpecially to all thoſe who are too weak to uſe any muſcular motion themſelves. A little friction may have little or no effect, but long con-tinued, and repeated often, with fumigated flannels, it will do more to recover health, and ſupport it afterwards, than moſt other things or methods. It promotes ciculation and perſpiration, opens the pores, forces the fine veſ-ſels, ſtrains and purifies the blood, and this without the aſſiſtance of any internal ſtimulation. It is this that keeps horſes in tolerable health with very litt'e exerciſe.

dare promife him fome amendment, & increafe of ftrength; which he muft employ, as young merchants do a little money, to get more. Thus he muft go on rubbing, walking, and riding a little more and more every day, ftopping always upon the firft fenfation of wearinefs to reft a little, till he be able to walk two or three miles at a ftretch, or ride ten without any wearinefs at all. This is recommended with an intention to diflodge and throw off all remains of crude gouty concretions that may have obftructed his joints, or lain concealed in any of the *lacunæ* or receffes of his body; to free the circulation *in minimis*, and all its fecretions, perfpirations, and difcharges whatever: and though this intention can never be but very defectively anfwered by medicines, it may certainly be affifted and greatly promoted by a few well-chofen mild antimonial, abforbent and faponaceous deobftruents and fweetners, that, like putting fhot or gravel into a bottle, with a good deal of agitation will greatly help to make it clean, but without agitation will do nothing *.

* The Afiatics, underftanding luxury much better than we do, and knowing that it is not to be had without fome degree of delicate health, do juft enough to keep them, in this languid effeminate ftate, free from pain. Thofe who are rich among them employ people called Champoers to rub, chafe, and pat them all over at leaft twice a day, to move their blood and keep their veffels free without any labor or exertion of their own powers. This daily practice in hot countries, where they live in the moft flothful indolence, is not only neceffary to them, but a great luxury. The Greeks and Romans too, when they became luxurious, fell into habits of this kind, and were ftrigilled, and curried, and bathed, and oiled, almoft every day.

While we are thus endeavoring to refolve all old obftructions, to open the fine veffels, and ftrain and purify the blood, and by degrees to enable the man to ule a certain degree of exercife or labor every day ; great care muft be taken in the choice of his diet, that no new acrimony be added to the old, to thwart and fruftrate this falutary operation. His food muft be foft, mild, and fpontaneoufly digefting, and in moderate quantity, fo as to give the leaft poffible labor to the ftomach and bowels ; that it may neither turn four, nor bitter, nor rancid, nor any way degenerate from thofe qualities neceffary to make good blood. Such things are, at firft, new-laid eggs boiled fo as not to harden the white creamy part of them, tripe, calves feet, chicken, partridge, rabbits, moft forts of white mild fifh, fuch as whiting, fkate, cod, turbot, &c. and all forts of fhell-fifh, particularly oyfters raw. Very foon he will be ftrong enough to eat beef, veal, mutton, lamb, pork, venifon, &c. but thefe muft all be kept till they are tender, and eaten with their own gravies without any compounded fauces or pickles whatever : inftead of which, boiled or ftewed vegetables, and fallads of lettuce and endive, may be ufed : and the luxury that is not unwholfome may be allowed, light puddings, cuftards, creams, blanc-manger, &c. and ripe fruits of all kinds and feafons. But becaufe * wine undoubt-

---

* I have made what inquiries I could upon this capital article from living witneffes ; for I do not always pin my faith upon books, knowing it to be no uncommon thing for authors, in ftead of framing their fyftem from obfervation and experience, to wreft and explain both to fupport their opinions. I have been affured by a phyfician who

edly produces nine in ten of all the gouts in the world, wine muſt be avoided, or taken very ſparingly, and but ſeldom. How is this to be done ? Can a man uſed to it every day, who thinks he cannot live without it, and that his exiſtence depends upon it, leave it off ſafely ? If he thinks he muſt die of the experiment, doing it all at once, he may do it by degrees, and drink but half the quantity of yeſterday till he has brought it to nothing. But the danger of attempting it in this manner is, that it will never be done ; and, like a procraſtinating ſinner, he will for ever put off his penitential reſolution till to-morrow. If he did it at all at once, I would be hanged if he died of the attempt ; he would be uneaſy for three or four days, that's all. He may change his liquor, and drink a little good porter, or ſoft ale, and by degrees come to ſmall beer, the wholſomeſt and beſt of all liquors except good ſoft water. I do not mean that this rigorous abſtinence from wine is to laſt for life, but only during the conflict with the diſeaſe. As ſoon as he has recovered health and ſtrength to uſe exerciſe enough to

practiſed above thirty years in Turkey, that from the Danube to the Euphrates he had never ſeen a gouty Turk. I have alſo been informed by ſome of our miniſters who had reſided many years at Conſtantinople, that the gout, and other diſeaſes of the ſame claſs, were not uncommon at court ; but the courtiers, it ſeems, were not as good Mahometans as thoſe who lived in the country ; for they drank wine, drams, liquors of all ſorts, without reſtraint.

I have alſo been very credibly informed, that the Gentoos or Marratas, a people of India living in the moſt temperate ſimplicity, chiefly upon rice, have no ſuch thing as the gout, or indeed any other chronic diſeaſe among them.

fubdue it, he may safely indulge once a week, or perhaps twice, with a point of wine for the fake of good humor and good company, if they cannot be enjoyed without it ; for I would not be such a churl as to forbid, or even damp, one of the greateſt joys of human life.

If any man ſhould fay, It is better to have a little gout than take all thefe pains, and fubmit. to this difcipline : this is not the alternative. Perhaps it may be more eligible to live at large, and have but a little gout now and then, that goes off well, and leaves no trace behind ; but this is very feldom the cafe. The misfortune is, that a little gout moſt commonly comes again and again more feverely, till it becomes a great gout, till it cripples the man, and ſhortens his life at leaſt twenty years, embittering all the latter part of it. If any one thinks this defcription of it, which is the real ſtate of the cafe nine times in ten, preferable to that gradual exertion of his own powers and ſtrictnefs of regimen, or rather attention to himfelf, with very moderate abſtinence or felf-denial for a year or two, as here recommended ; I have no reply to make him, but muſt give him up to his own choice.

The feverity of thefe efforts, and this abſtemious care need be continued no longer than the difeafe or the effects of it remain. When by prefeverance in the practice of them, together with the medical aids here recommended, the patient ſhall have recovered his strength and locomotive powers, he may preserve and perpetuate them, and make good his title to longevity, upon the following plan.

He must never lose sight of the three great principles of health and long life, Activity, Temperance, & Peace of Mind. With these ever in view, he may eat and drink of every thing the earth produces, but his diet must be plain, simple, solid and tender, or in proportion to his consumption ; he must eat but of one thing or two at most at a meal, and this will soon bring him to be satisfied with about half his usual quantity ; for all men eat about twice as much as they ought to do, provoked by variety : he must drink but little of any liquor, and never till he has done eating : the drier every man's diet is, the better. No wine oftener than once or twice a week at most ; and this must be considered as a luxurious indulgence. If he be sometimes led unawares into a debauch, it must be expiated by abstinence and double exercise the next day, and he may take a little of my magnesia and rhubarb as a good antidote : or if he cannot sleep with his unusual load, he may drink water, and with his finger in his throat throw it up. I have known some old soldiers by this trick alone, never taking their dose to bed with them, live to kill their acquaintance two or three times over. One moderate meal a day is abundantly sufficient ; therefore it is better to omit supper, because dinner is not so easily avoided. Instead of supper, any good ripe fruit of the season would be very salutary, preventing costiveness, and keeping the bowels free and open, cooling, correcting, and carrying off the heats and crudities of his indigeftion.

His activity need be no more than to perfevere in the habit of rubbing all over night and morning for eight or ten minutes, and walking three or four miles every day, or riding ten, or ufing any bodily labor or exercife equivalent to it. In bad weather I can fee no great evil in throwing a cloak round his fhoulders and walking even in the rain ; the only difficulty is to fummon refolution enough to venture out ; and a little ufe would take off all danger of catching cold, by hardening and fecuring him a-gainft the poffibility of it upon that and all other occafions. If he dares not rifque this, fome fucce-daneum muft be ufed within doors ; more efpecially when bad weather continues any time. I recom-mend it to all men to wafh their feet every day, the gouty in particular, and not lie a-bed above feven hours in fummer, and eight in winter.

Whoever thinks there cannot be luxury enough in this courfe of life, I am perfuaded will not find more in any other : for good health, with all it's natural appetites and fenfations in perfect order, is the only true foundation of luxury. And whoever cultivates it upon the falfe principles of culinary or medical art, urging to excefs by ftimulating provo-catives of any kind, inftead of pleafure and enjoy-ment, will meet with pain and difguft.

Some perhaps may be reafonable enough to obferve and fay, This plan of yours is very fimple ;
there is nothing marvellous in it ; no wonderful
difcovery of any of the latent powers of medicine :
but will a regimen, fo eafy to be comply'd with as
this cure the gout, ftone, dropfy, &c. ? Will it repair broken conftitutions and reftore old invalids to
health ? My anfwer is, that if I may truft the experience of my whole life, and above all the experience I have had in my own perfon, having not
only got rid of the gout, of which I have had four
fevere fits in my younger days, but alfo emerged
from the loweft ebb of life, that a man could poffibly be reduced to by colic, jaundice, and a complication of complaints, and recovered to perfect
health ; which I have now uninterruptedly enjoyed
above ten years : I fay, if I may rely upon all this,
I may with great fafety pronounce and promife that
the plan here recommended, affifted at firft with all
the collateral aids of medicine peculiar to each cafe,
correcting many an untoward concomitant fymptom,
purfued with refolution and patience, will certainly
procure to others the fame benefits I received from
it, and cure every curable difeafe. If this be thought
too much to promife, I beg it may be confidered,
that a life of bad habits produces all thefe difeafes :
nothing therefore fo likely as good ones long continued to reftore or preferve health.

What can the beft phyfician do more than difco-
ver and point out to his patients the real caufes of

their difeafes ? You will fay, he muſt find a remedy: this he will do for you alfo as long as he can. But I will tell you a fecret: his remedies are chiefly evacuations ; as long as your body can bear fcouring and cleanfing,* he will do you fome temporary apparent fervice : but when it begins to wear out, his remedies will anfwer no longer ; you muſt try better methods ; you muſt not repeat the caufe fo often ; for he cannot for ever build up as faſt as you can pull down. In fhort, you muſt reform your life, and change all your bad habits for good ones ; and if you have patience to wait the flow operations of nature properly affiſted, you will have no reafon to regret your former luxuries.

We are all fo much the creatures of habit, which forms and fafhions us to good or ill almoſt as much as nature itfelf, that we ought to be very attentive and careful that our daily habits may ever tend to the confirmation, not the deftruction of health. It is not what we do now and then that can injure us greatly, but what we do every day muſt either do us great good or harm ; either eftablifhing our health, or fixing our difeafes, for life.

* Paracelfus was a good chemiſt, but a miferable phyfician : he invented the medicine which he moſt ridiculoufly called *Elixir proprietatis* ; and from it's efficacy, fot as he was, promifed himfelf the years of Methufalem. At firſt it did wonders, fcoured and carried off all his crapulary indigeſtions, and kept him fome time in health and fpirits ; but trufting to it too long, and repeating it too often, it not only loft all it's power of doing good, but hurt him greatly, and he died, I think, at fix-and-thirty, notwithſtanding his Elixir.

If, after all, any man fhould fay, thefe reftraints, this care in chufing what is wholfome, this conftant watching over all we do, would make life fo grievous, that health were not worth having upon thefe terms ; I wifh him to ftop a little, and confider them well before he rejects them in tirely ; and whether there be any better for him. It can do him no great harm to try a month or two ; if he does I flatter myfelf he will find that cuftom will take off the greateft part of the grievance, and perfeverance make them not only tolerable but pleafant. If he thinks health may be enjoyed upo eafier terms, I fear he will be miferably deceived ; for health like beauty, may be won by our own attention,efforts, and affiduities, but cannot be had by purchafe. Whoever thinks to buy either, will have the misfortune to find it not long his own, though he has paid for it.

But there may be others whom long fuffe ring has made more patient and reafonable : thefe may be glad to hear that a little health is to be had on any terms ; and it may be very comfortable to them to know that there is fcarcely any ftate of weaknefs fo low, fuppofing the vitals not mortally hurt,from which they may not recover into very defirable health & ftrength, & by thefe means,exerted with perfevering patience. I fay this to invalids in general : for thus may be cured not only the gout, but very bad rheumatifms, ifchiaticas, rickets, ftone, jaundice, dropfy, afthma, cachexies, and complications of many kind ; not excepting even cancers, if they are not too far gone :

for a cancer is nothing more than a place where nature depofits the bad humors of the blood, as appears by its almoft conftant return to fome other part after extirpation. Whatever chronic difeafe will not give way to this fyftem of medication, will be found, I greatly fear, too hard for any other. And fhould there be a particular cafe, in which fome fortunate violence or chance may have apparently fucceeded for a time, the return of the evil, or change to fomething worfe, can no way be fo well guarded againft and prevented, as by fome rational and natural inftitution of life.

Thus have I endeavored to fet forth the real caufes of chronic difeafes in general and the true principles of convalefcence, health, and longevity. If I have hazarded any thing new, or contrary to received opinions, it has been from a thorough conviction of it's truth, however dangerous to fame and fortune ; both which I know are more eafily acquired by complying with the world, than attempting to reform it : but it muft be fomebody equally indifferent to both, as I am, who will venture to tell fuch truths as are more likely to recoil and hurt the author, than to convince and conciliate the bulk of mankind.

T H E   E N D.

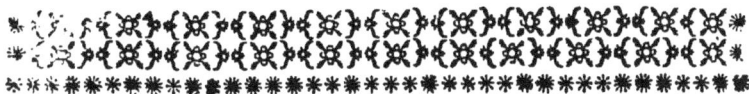

LONDON BOOK-STORE, a little Southward of
the Town-Houfe, in Cornhill, *Bofton*,

HENRY KNOX,

Imports and fells BOOKS in all Languages, Arts,
andSciences, either by Wholefale or Retail ;——
Some of which are the following much efteemed
Authors in Phyfic and Surgery,

AITKIN's Effays on feveral important Subjects
in Surgery, with Plates, 8vo.
Aikin's Obfervations on the external Ufe of Prepa
rations of Lead.
Aikin's Thoughts on Hofpitals.
Brookes's Introduction to Phyfic and Surgery, 8vo.
———— Practice of Phyfic, 2 vol. 8vo.
Buckner's Effay and Practicable Method to enable
Deaf Perfons to hear.
Chapman's Midwifery 8vo.
Chefleden's Anatomy.
Caverhill's Experiments of the Caufes of Heat in
living Animals.
Edinburgh Difpenfatory, 8vo.
Elfe on the Hydrocele.,
Fordyce's Practice of Phyfic, 8vo.
————— On the Venereal Difeafe.

Grant's Enquiry into the Nature and Progress of Fevers, with Obfervations on the beft Method of treating them, 8vo.

Haller's Phifiology, 2 vol. 8vo.

———— On Irratibility.

Hill's Family Herbal.

Huxham on Fevers.

———— On Antimony.

Hunter's elegant Treatife on the Teeth, withPlates, 4to.

James's Difpenfatory, 8vo.

———— On Canine Madnefs.

Lobb's Practice of Phyfic, 2 vol.

Lind on Difeafes incident to Europeans in Hot Climates, 8vo.

LeDran's Operations in Surgery, 8vo.

Langrifh's Practice of Phyfic, 8vo.

Monro on the Dropfy.

Mead's Medical Precepts and Cautions.

MacBride's Experimental Effays on Medical and Philofophical Subjects, 8vo.

McKenzie on Health, 8vo.

Medical Obfervations and Inquiries by a Society of Phyficians in London, 4 vol. 8vo.

The 4th vol. may be had fingle.

Millar on the Afthma and Hooping Cough, 8vo.

Manning on Female Difeafes, 8vo.

Medulla Medicinæ Univerfæ, 12mo.

Northcote's Marine Practice of Phyfic, 2 vol. 8vo.

Pott on the Hydrocele,

Pemberton's Difpenfatory.

Practice of the London Hofpitals

Quincy's Difpenfatory, 8vo.
———— Lexicon, 8vo.
Roupe on the Difeafes of Seamen.
Rowley's Effay on the Ophthalmia.
———— ·——— On the Cure of Ulcerated Legs with-
out reft.
Shaw's Practice of Phyfic, 2 vol.
Tiffot on Health.
——— On Onanifm.
——— On Difeafes incident to literary and fedentary
Perfons.
Wilfon's Chemiftry, 8vo.
Winflow's Anatomy, 4to.
White's Cafes in Surgery, with Plates. 8vo. &c. &c.

www.ingramcontent.com/pod-product-compliance
Lightning Source LLC
Chambersburg PA
CBHW022142090426
42742CB00010B/1353